Anti

inflammatory diet cookbook for beginners

The complete cookbook for beginners, lose up to 5 pounds in 7 days with amazing and flavourful recipes.

Joseph Monroe

Legal & Disclaimer

The information contained in this book and its contents is not designed to replace or take the place of any form of medical or professional advice; and is not meant to replace the need for independent medical, financial, legal or other professional advice or services, as may be required. The content and information in this book have been provided for educational and entertainment purposes only.

The content and information contained in this book have been compiled from sources deemed reliable, and it is accurate to the best of the Author's knowledge, information, and belief. However, the author cannot guarantee its accuracy and validity and cannot be held liable for any errors and/or omissions. Further, changes are periodically made to this book as and when needed. Where appropriate and/or necessary, you must consult a professional (including but not limited to your doctor, attorney, financial advisor or such other professional advisor) before using any of the suggested remedies, techniques, or information in this book.

Upon using the contents and information contained in this book, you agree to hold harmless the Author from and against any damages, costs, and expenses, including any legal fees potentially resulting from the application of any of the information provided by this book. This disclaimer applies to any loss, damages or injury caused by the use and application, whether directly or indirectly, of any advice or information presented, whether for breach of contract, tort, negligence, personal injury, criminal intent, or under any other cause of action.

You agree to accept all risks of using the information presented inside this book.

You agree that by continuing to read this book, where appropriate and/or necessary, you shall consult a professional (including but not limited to your doctor, attorney, or financial advisor or such other advisor as needed) before using any of the suggested remedies, techniques, or information in this book.

TABLE OF CONTENTS

SIDE DISHES   44

BREAKFAST

1. Raspberry Steel Cut Oatmeal Bars

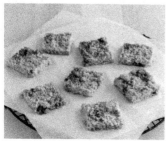

Preparation Time: 5 minutes
Cooking Time: 15 minutes
Servings: 6

Ingredients:

- 3 cups steel cut oats
- 3 large eggs
- 2 cups unsweetened vanilla almond milk
- 1/3 cup erythritol
- 1 teaspoon pure vanilla extract
- ¼ teaspoon salt
- 1 cup frozen raspberries

Directions:

1. In a medium bowl, mix together all ingredients except the raspberries. Once the ingredients are well combined, fold in the raspberries.
2. Spray a 6" cake pan with cooking oil. Transfer the oat mixture to the pan and cover the pan with aluminum foil.
3. Pour 1 cup water into the Instant Pot® and place the steam rack inside. Place the pan with the oat mixture on top of the rack. Secure the lid.

4. Press the Manual or Pressure Cook button and adjust the time to 15 minutes.
5. When the timer beeps, quick-release pressure until float valve drops and then unlock lid.
6. Carefully remove the pan from the inner pot and remove the foil. Allow to cool completely before cutting into bars and serving.

Nutrition: Calories: 399 | Fat: 9g | Protein: 18g | Sodium: 192mg Fiber: 12g | Carbohydrates: 72g | Sugar: 1g

2. Blueberry Vanilla Quinoa Porridge

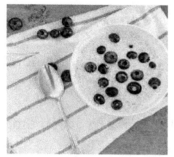

Preparation Time: 2 minutes
Cooking Time: 1 minute
Servings: 6

Ingredients:

- 1½ cups dry quinoa
- 3 cups water
- 1 cup frozen wild blueberries
- ½ teaspoon pure stevia powder
- 1 teaspoon pure vanilla extract

Directions:

1. Using a fine-mesh strainer, rinse the quinoa very well until the water runs clear.
2. Add the quinoa, water, blueberries, stevia, and vanilla to the inner pot. Stir to combine. Secure the lid.
3. Press the Manual or Pressure Cook button and adjust the time to 1 minute.
4. When the timer beeps, quick-release pressure until float valve drops and then unlock lid.
5. Allow the quinoa to cool slightly before spooning into bowls to serve.

Nutrition: Calories: 181 | Fat: 3g | Protein: 6g | Sodium: 9mg Fiber: 5g | Carbohydrates: 33g | Sugar: 3g

3. Buckwheat Ginger Granola

Preparation Time: 10 minutes
Cooking Time: 10 minutes
Servings: 8

Ingredients:

- 1½ cups raw buckwheat groats
- 1½ cups old fashioned rolled oats
- 1/3 cup walnuts, coarsely chopped
- 1/3 cup unsweetened shredded coconut
- ¼ cup coconut oil, melted
- 1"-piece fresh ginger, peeled and grated
- 3 tablespoons date syrup
- 1 teaspoon ground cinnamon
- ¼ teaspoon salt

Directions:

1. In a medium bowl, mix together the buckwheat groats, oats, walnuts, and shredded coconut until well combined. Add the coconut oil, ginger, date syrup, cinnamon, and salt and stir to combine.
2. Transfer this mixture to a 6" cake pan.
3. Pour 1 cup water into the inner pot and place a steam rack inside. Place the pan on the rack. Secure the lid.
4. Press the Manual or Pressure Cook button and adjust the time to 10 minutes.
5. When the timer beeps, quick-release pressure until float valve drops and then unlock lid.
6. Spread the granola onto a large sheet pan and allow it to cool, undisturbed, for 1 hour. It will crisp as it cools.

Nutrition: Calories: 311 | Fat: 13g | Protein: 7g | Sodium: 78mg Fiber: 6g | Carbohydrates: 42g | Sugar: 6g

4. Coconut Chocolate Oatmeal

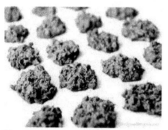

Preparation Time: 5 minutes
Cooking Time: 6 minutes
Servings: 4

Ingredients:

- 1 cup steel cut oats
- 1 (13.25-ounce) can full-fat unsweetened coconut milk
- 2 cups water
- ½ cup cacao powder
- ½ cup erythritol
- 1/8 teaspoon sea salt

Directions:

1. Place the oats, coconut milk, water, cacao powder, erythritol, and salt in the inner pot and stir to combine. Secure the lid.
2. Press the Manual or Pressure Cook button and adjust the time to 6 minutes.
3. When the timer beeps, quick-release pressure until float valve drops and then unlock lid.
4. Allow the oatmeal to cool slightly before spooning into bowls to serve.

Nutrition: Calories: 394 | Fat: 23g | Protein: 11g | Sodium: 60mg Fiber: 7g | Carbohydrates: 62g | Sugar: 0g

5. Banana Date Porridge

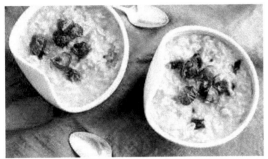

Preparation Time: 5 minutes
Cooking Time: 4 minutes
Servings: 4

Ingredients:

- 1 cup buckwheat groats
- 1½ cups unsweetened vanilla almond milk
- 1 cup water
- 1 large banana, mashed
- 5 pitted dates, chopped
- ¾ teaspoon ground cinnamon
- ¾ teaspoon pure vanilla extract

Directions:

1. Place the buckwheat groats, almond milk, water, banana, dates, cinnamon, and vanilla in the inner pot and stir. Secure the lid.
2. Press the Manual or Pressure Cook button and adjust the time to 4 minutes.
3. When the timer beeps, quick-release pressure until float valve drops and then unlock lid.
4. Allow the porridge to cool slightly before spooning into bowls to serve.

Nutrition: Calories: 211 | Fat: 2g | Protein: 6g | Sodium: 72mg Fiber: 6g | Carbohydrates: 46g | Sugar: 10g

6. Banana Baked Oatmeal

Preparation Time: 5 minutes
Cooking Time: 7 minutes
Servings: 6

Ingredients:

- 3 cups old fashioned rolled oats
- ¼ teaspoon salt
- 2 large bananas, mashed (1 heaping cup)
- 2 large eggs, lightly beaten
- 1/3 cup xylitol

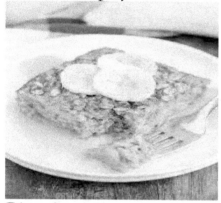

Directions:

1. In a medium bowl, place the oats, salt, bananas, eggs, and xylitol and stir to combine well.
2. Lightly spray a 6" cake pan with cooking spray. Transfer the oat mixture to the pan.
3. Pour 1½ cups water into the inner pot. Place a steam rack in the inner pot and place the pan on the steam rack. Secure the lid.
4. Press the Manual or Pressure Cook button and adjust the time to 7 minutes.
5. When the timer beeps, quick-release pressure until float valve drops and then unlock lid.
6. Allow the oatmeal to cool 5 minutes before serving.

Nutrition: Calories: 280 | Fat: 5g | Protein: 10g | Sodium: 120mg Fiber: 6g | Carbohydrates: 53g | Sugar: 7g

7. Banana Walnut Steel Cut Oats

Preparation Time: 2 minutes
Cooking Time: 4 minutes
Servings: 4

Ingredients:

- 2 cups steel cut oats
- 2½ cups water
- 2½ cups unsweetened vanilla almond milk
- 3 medium bananas, thinly sliced
- 1½ teaspoons ground cinnamon
- 1 teaspoon pure vanilla extract
- ¼ teaspoon salt
- 4 tablespoons walnut pieces

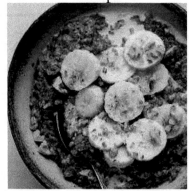

Directions:

1. Add the steel cut oats, water, almond milk, banana slices, cinnamon, vanilla, and salt to the Instant Pot® and stir to combine. Secure the lid.
2. Press the Manual or Pressure Cook button on the Instant Pot® and adjust the time to 4 minutes.
3. When the timer beeps, let pressure release naturally for 15 minutes, then quick-release any remaining pressure until float valve drops, then unlock lid.

4. Serve the oatmeal in a bowl topped with 1 tablespoon walnut pieces for each serving.

Nutrition: Calories: 491 | Fat: 13g | Protein: 17g | Sodium: 258mg Fiber: 14g | Carbohydrates: 81g | Sugar: 11g

8. Spinach and Artichoke Egg Casserole

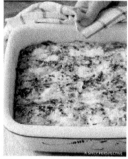

Preparation Time: 10 minutes
Cooking Time: 18 minutes
Servings: 8

Ingredients:

- 12 large eggs
- ¼ cup water
- 4 cups baby spinach, roughly chopped
- 1 (14-ounce) can baby artichoke hearts, drained and roughly chopped
- 1 tablespoon chopped fresh chives
- 1 tablespoon fresh lemon juice
- ¾ teaspoon table salt
- ½ teaspoon black pepper
- ¼ teaspoon garlic salt

Directions:

1. Spray a 6" round pan or 7-cup round glass bowl with cooking spray.
2. In a medium bowl, whisk together the eggs and water.
3. Stir in the spinach, artichokes, chives, lemon juice, table salt, pepper, and garlic salt.
4. Transfer the mixture to the prepared pan.

5. Place 2 cups water in the inner pot and place the steam rack inside. Place the pan on top of the steam rack. Secure the lid.
6. Press the Manual or Pressure Cook button and adjust the time to 18 minutes.
7. When the timer beeps, quick-release pressure until float valve drops and then unlock lid.
8. Remove egg casserole from pot and allow to cool 5 minutes before slicing and serving.

Nutrition: Calories: 122 | Fat: 7g | Protein: 10g | Sodium: 603mg Fiber: 1g | Carbohydrates: 3g | Sugar: 1g

9. Coconut Almond Granola

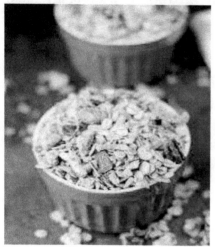

Preparation Time: 5 minutes
Cooking Time: 7 minutes
Servings: 8

Ingredients:

- 1½ cups old fashioned rolled oats
- ½ cup unsweetened shredded coconut
- ¼ cup monk fruit sweetener
- 1/8 teaspoon salt
- ¾ cup almond butter
- ¼ cup coconut oil

Directions:

1. In a medium bowl, mix together the oats, coconut, sweetener, and salt. Add the almond butter and oil and mix until well combined.
2. Spray a 6" cake pan with nonstick cooking oil. Transfer the oat mixture to the pan.
3. Add 1 cup water to the inner pot of your Instant Pot®. Place the steam rack inside, and place the pan on top of the steam rack. Secure the lid.

4. Press the Manual or Pressure Cook button and adjust the time to 7 minutes.
5. When the timer beeps, quick-release pressure until float valve drops and then unlock lid.
6. Remove the pan from the inner pot and transfer the granola to a baking sheet to cool completely (at least 30 minutes) before serving.

Nutrition: Calories: 307 | Fat: 22g | Protein: 8g | Sodium: 37mg Fiber: 5g | Carbohydrates: 24g | Sugar: 2g

10. Pumpkin Quinoa Porridge

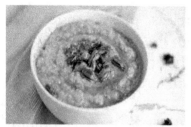

Preparation Time: 2 minutes
Cooking Time: 1 minute
Servings: 4

Ingredients:

- ¾ cup dry quinoa
- 2 cups water
- ¾ cup pumpkin purée
- ¼ cup monk fruit sweetener
- 1½ teaspoons pumpkin pie spice
- 1 teaspoon pure vanilla extract
- ¼ teaspoon salt
1. Using a fine-mesh strainer, rinse the quinoa very well until the water runs clear.

Add the quinoa, water, pumpkin purée, sweetener, pumpkin pie spice, vanilla, and salt to the inner pot. Stir to **Directions:**

2. combine. Secure the lid.
3. Press the Manual or Pressure Cook button and adjust the time to 1 minute.
4. When the timer beeps, quick-release pressure until float valve drops and then unlock lid.
5. Allow the quinoa to cool slightly before spooning into bowls to serve.

Nutrition: Calories: 141 | Fat: 2g | Protein: 5g | Sodium: 148mg Fiber: 3g | Carbohydrates: 37g | Sugar: 2g

LUNCH

11. Roasted Brussels Sprouts & Sweet Potato

Preparation Time: 15 minutes
Cooking Time: 45 minutes
Servings: 6-8
Ingredients:
- 1 large sweet potato, peeled and cut into 1-2-nch pieces
- 1 pound Brussels sprouts, trimmed and halved
- 2 minced garlic cloves
- 1 teaspoon ground cumin
- ½ teaspoon garlic salt
- Salt and freshly ground black pepper, to taste
- 1/3 cup olive oil
- 1 tablespoon apple cider vinegar
- Chopped fresh thyme, for garnishing

Directions:
1. Preheat the oven to 400 degrees F. Grease a sheet pan.
2. In a large bowl, add all ingredients except vinegar and thyme and toss to coat well.
3. Transfer the mixture into prepared baking pan.
4. Roast for 40-45 minutes more.
5. Transfer the vegetable mixture in a serving plate and drizzle with vinegar.
6. Garnish with thyme and serve.

Nutrition: Calories: 127 kcal Protein: 2.48 g Fat: 9.18 g Carbohydrates: 10.38 g

12. Potato Mash

Preparation Time: 15 minutes
Cooking Time: 20 minutes
Servings: 32

Ingredients:

- 10 large baking potatoes, peeled and cubed
- 3 tablespoons olive oil, divided
- 1 onion, chopped
- 1 tablespoon ground turmeric
- ½ teaspoon ground cumin
- Salt and freshly ground black pepper, to taste

Directions:

1. In a large pan of water, add potatoes and bring to a boil on medium-high heat.
2. Cook for about 20 minutes.
3. Drain well and transfer into a large bowl.
4. With a potato masher, mash the potatoes.
5. Meanwhile in a skillet, heat 1 tablespoon of oil on medium-high heat.
6. Add onion and sauté for about 6 minutes.
7. Add onion mixture into the bowl with mashed potatoes.
8. Add turmeric, cumin, salt and black pepper and mash till well combined.
9. Stir in remaining oil and serve.

Nutrition Calories: 103 Fat: 4g Sat Fat: 2g Carbohydrates: 23g Fiber: 2g Sugar: 1g Protein: 8g Sodium: 224mg

13. Creamy Sweet Potato Mash

Preparation Time: 15 minutes
Cooking Time: 21 minutes
Servings: 4

Ingredients:
- 1 tbsp. olive oil
- 2 large sweet potatoes, peeled and chopped
- 2 teaspoons ground turmeric
- 1 garlic clove, minced
- 2 cups vegetable broth
- 2 tablespoons unsweetened coconut milk
- Salt and freshly ground black pepper, to taste
- Chopped pistachios, for garnishing

Directions:
1. In a large skillet, heat oil on medium-high heat.
2. Add sweet potato and stir fry for bout 2-3 minutes.
3. Add turmeric and stir fry for about 1 minute.
4. Add garlic and stir fry for about 2 minutes.
5. Add broth and bring to a boil.
6. Reduce the heat to low and cook for about 10-15 minutes or till all the liquid is absorbed.
7. Transfer the sweet potato mixture into a bowl.
8. Add coconut milk, salt and black pepper and mash it completely.
9. Garnish with pistachio and serve.

Nutrition Calories: 110 Fat: 5g Carbohydrates: 16g Protein: 1g

14. Gingered Cauliflower Rice

Preparation Time: 15 minutes
Cooking Time: 10 minutes
Servings: 3-4

Ingredients:

- 3 tablespoons coconut oil
- 4 (1/8-inch thick) fresh ginger slices
- 1 small head cauliflower, trimmed and processed into rice consistency
- 3 garlic cloves, crushed
- 1 tablespoon chives, chopped
- 1 tablespoon coconut vinegar
- Salt, to taste

Directions:

1. In a skillet, melt coconut oil on medium-high heat.
2. Add ginger and sauté for about 2-3 minutes.
3. Discard the ginger slices and stir in cauliflower and garlic.
4. Cook, stirring occasionally for about 7-8 minutes.
5. Stir in remaining ingredients and remove from heat.
6. Serve immediately

Nutrition: Calories: 111 kcal Protein: 1.48 g Fat: 10.42 g Carbohydrates: 4.49 g

15. Spicy Cauliflower Rice

Preparation Time: 15 minutes
Cooking Time: 10 minutes
Servings: 4
Ingredients:

- 3 tablespoons coconut oil
- 1 small white onion, chopped
- 3 garlic cloves, minced
- 1 large head cauliflower, trimmed and processed into rice consistency
- ½ teaspoon ground cumin
- ½ teaspoon paprika
- Salt and freshly ground black pepper, to taste
- 1large tomato, chopped
- ¼ cup tomato paste
- ¼ cup fresh cilantro, chopped
- Chopped fresh cilantro, for garnishing
- 2 limes, quarters

Directions:

1. In a large skillet, melt coconut oil on medium-high heat.
2. Add onion and sauté for about 2 minutes.
3. Add garlic and sauté for about 1 minute.
4. Stir in cauliflower rice.
5. Add cumin, paprika, salt and black pepper and cook, stirring occasionally for about 2-3 minutes.
6. Stir in tomato, tomato paste and cilantro and cook for about 2-3 minutes.
7. Garnish with cilantro and serve alongside lime.

Nutrition: Calories: 137 kcal Protein: 2.73 g Fat: 10.69 g Carbohydrates: 11.1 g

16. Simple Brown Rice

Preparation Time: 10 minutes
Cooking Time: 50 minutes
Servings: 4
Ingredients:
- 1 cup brown rice
- 2 cups chicken broth
- 1 tablespoon ground turmeric
- 1 tbsp. olive oil

Directions:
1. In a pan, add rice, broth and turmeric and bring to a boil.
2. Reduce the heat to low.
3. Simmer, covered for about 50 minutes.
4. Add the olive oil and fluff with a fork.
5. Keep aside, covered for about 10 minutes before serving.

Nutrition: Calories: 227 kcal Protein: 26.16 g Fat: 11.75 g Carbohydrates: 2.5 g

17. Quinoa with Apricots

Preparation Time: 15 minutes
Cooking Time: 12 minutes
Servings: 4
Ingredients:

- 2 cups water
- 1 cup quinoa
- ½ teaspoon fresh ginger, grated finely
- ½ cup dried apricots, chopped roughly
- Salt and freshly ground black pepper, to taste

Directions:

1. In a pan, add water on high heat and bring to a boil.
2. Add quinoa and reduce the heat to medium.
3. Cover and reduce the heat to low.
4. Simmer for about 12 minutes.
5. Remove from heat and immediately, stir in ginger and apricots.
6. Keep aside, covered for about 15 minutes before serving.

Nutrition: Calories: 196 kcal Protein: 6.56 g Fat: 2.66 g Carbohydrates: 37.49 g

18. Simple Carrots Mix

Preparation time: ten minutes
Cooking time: 40 minutes
Servings: 6
Ingredients:
- 15 carrots, halved lengthwise
- 2 tablespoons coconut sugar
- ¼ cup extra virgin organic olive oil
- ½ teaspoon rosemary, dried
- ½ teaspoon garlic powder
- A pinch of black pepper

Directions:
1. In a bowl, combine the carrots with the sugar, oil, rosemary, garlic powder and black pepper, toss well, spread with a lined baking sheet, introduce in the oven and bake at 400 degrees F for 40 minutes.
2. Divide between plates and serve as a side dish.
3. Enjoy!

Nutrition: calories 211, fat 2, fiber 6, carbs 14, protein 8

19. Tasty Grilled Asparagus

Preparation time: 10 minutes
Cooking time: 6 minutes
Servings: 4

Ingredients:

- 2 pounds asparagus, trimmed
- 2 tablespoons organic olive oil
- A pinch of salt and black pepper

Directions:

1. In a bowl, combine the asparagus with salt, pepper and oil and toss well.
2. Place the asparagus on preheated grill over medium-high heat, cook for 3 minutes with them, divide between plates and serve as being a side dish.
3. Enjoy!

Nutrition: calories 172, fat 4, fiber 7, carbs 14, protein 8

20. Easy Roasted Carrots

Preparation time: ten mins
Cooking time: 30 minutes
Servings: 4

Ingredients:
- 2 pounds carrots, quartered
- A pinch of black pepper
- 3 tablespoons olive oil
- 2 tablespoons parsley, chopped

Directions:
1. Arrange the carrots with a lined baking sheet, add black pepper and oil, toss, introduce inside the oven and cook at 400 degrees F to get a half-hour.
2. Add parsley, toss, divide between plates and serve as a side dish.
3. Enjoy!

Nutrition: calories 177, fat 3, fiber 6, carbs 14, protein 6

DINNER

21. Garlicky Chicken and Vegetables

Preparation Time: 10 minutes
Cooking Time: 45 minutes
Servings: 4

Ingredients:

- 2 teaspoons extra-virgin olive oil
- 1 leek, white part only, thinly sliced
- 2 large zucchinis, cut into ¼-inch slices
- 4 bone-in, skin-on chicken breasts
- 3 garlic cloves, minced
- 1 teaspoon salt
- 1 teaspoon dried oregano
- ¼ teaspoon freshly ground black pepper
- ½ cup white wine
- Juice of 1 lemon

Directions:

1. Preheat the oven to 400°F. Grease the baking sheet with the oil.
2. Place the leek and zucchini on the baking sheet.
3. Put the chicken, skin-side up, and sprinkle with the garlic, salt, oregano, and pepper. Add the wine.
4. Roast within 35 to 40 minutes. Remove and let rest for 5 minutes.
5. Add the lemon juice and serve.

Nutrition: Calories: 315 Total Fat: 8g Total Carbohydrates: 12g Sugar: 4g Fiber: 2g Protein: 44g Sodium: 685mg

22. Turmeric-Spiced Sweet Potatoes, Apple, and Onion with Chicken

Preparation Time: 15 minutes
Cooking Time: 45 minutes
Servings: 4

Ingredients:

- 2 tablespoons unsalted butter, at room temperature
- 2 medium sweet potatoes
- 1 large Granny Smith apple
- 1 medium onion, thinly sliced
- 4 bone-in, skin-on chicken breasts
- 1 teaspoon salt
- 1 teaspoon turmeric
- 1 teaspoon dried sage
- ¼ teaspoon freshly ground black pepper
- 1 cup apple cider, white wine, or chicken broth

Directions:

1. Preheat the oven to 400°F. Grease the baking sheet with the butter.
2. Arrange the sweet potatoes, apple, and onion in a single layer on the baking sheet.
3. Put the chicken, skin-side up, and season with the salt, turmeric, sage, and pepper. Add the cider.
4. Roast within 35 to 40 minutes. Remove, let it rest for 5 minutes and serve.

Nutrition: Calories: 386 Total Fat: 12g Total Carbohydrates: 26g Sugar: 10g Fiber: 4g Protein: 44g Sodium: 932mg

23. Honey-Roasted Chicken Thighs with Carrots

Preparation Time: 10 minutes
Cooking Time: 50 minutes
Servings: 4

Ingredients:

- 2 tablespoons unsalted butter, at room temperature
- 3 large carrots, thinly sliced
- 2 garlic cloves, minced
- 4 bone-in, skin-on chicken thighs
- 1 teaspoon salt
- ½ teaspoon dried rosemary
- ¼ teaspoon freshly ground black pepper
- 2 tablespoons honey
- 1 cup chicken broth or vegetable broth
- Lemon wedges, for serving

Directions:

1. Preheat the oven to 400°F. Grease the baking sheet with the butter.
2. Arrange the carrots and garlic in a single layer on the baking sheet.
3. Put the chicken, skin-side up, on top of the vegetables, and season with the salt, rosemary, and pepper.
4. Put the honey on top and add the broth.
5. Roast within 40 to 45 minutes. Remove, and then let it rest for 5 minutes, and serve with lemon wedges.

Nutrition: Calories: 428 Total Fat: 28g Total Carbohydrates: 15g Sugar: 11g Fiber: 2g Protein: 30g Sodium: 732mg

24. Sesame-Tamari Baked Chicken with Green Beans

Preparation Time: 10 minutes
Cooking Time: 45 minutes
Servings: 4

Ingredients:

- 1-pound green beans, trimmed
- 4 bone-in, skin-on chicken breasts
- 2 tablespoons honey
- 1 tablespoon sesame oil
- 1 tablespoon gluten-free tamari or soy sauce
- 1 cup chicken or vegetable broth

Directions:

1. Preheat the oven to 400°F.
2. Arrange the green beans on a large rimmed baking sheet.
3. Put the chicken, skin-side up, on top of the beans.
4. Drizzle with the honey, oil, and tamari. Add the broth.
5. Roast within 35 to 40 minutes. Remove, let it rest for 5 minutes and serve.

Nutrition: Calories: 378 Total Fat: 10g Total Carbohydrates: 19g Sugar: 10g Fiber: 4g Protein: 54g Sodium: 336mg

25. Sheet Pan Turkey Breast with Golden Vegetables

Preparation Time: 15 minutes
Cooking Time: 45 minutes
Servings: 4

Ingredients:

- 2 tablespoons unsalted butter, at room temperature
- 1 medium acorn squash, seeded and thinly sliced
- 2 large golden beets, peeled and thinly sliced
- ½ medium yellow onion, thinly sliced
- ½ boneless, skin-on turkey breast (1 to 2 pounds)
- 2 tablespoons honey
- 1 teaspoon salt
- 1 teaspoon turmeric
- ¼ teaspoon freshly ground black pepper
- 1 cup chicken broth or vegetable broth

Directions:

1. Preheat the oven to 400°F. Grease the baking sheet with the butter.
2. Arrange the squash, beets, and onion in a single layer on the baking sheet. Put the turkey skin-side up. Drizzle with the honey. Season with the salt, turmeric, and pepper, and add the broth.
3. Roast until the turkey registers 165°F in the center with an instant-read thermometer, 35 to 45 minutes. Remove, and let rest for 5 minutes.
4. Slice, and serve.

Nutrition: Calories: 383 Total Fat: 15g Total Carbohydrates: 25g Sugar: 13g Fiber: 3g Protein: 37g Sodium: 748mg

26. Sheet Pan Steak with Brussels sprouts And Red Wine

Preparation Time: 10 minutes
Cooking Time: 20 minutes
Servings: 4

Ingredients:

- 1-pound rib-eye steak
- 1 teaspoon salt
- ¼ teaspoon freshly ground black pepper
- 1 tablespoon unsalted butter
- ½ red onion, minced
- 8 ounces Brussels sprouts, trimmed and quartered
- 1 cup red wine
- Juice of ½ lemon

Directions:

1. Preheat the broiler on high.
2. Massage the steak with the salt and pepper on a large rimmed baking sheet. Broil until browned, 2 to 3 minutes per side.
3. Turn off and heat-up the oven to 400°F.
4. Put the steak on one side of the baking sheet and add the butter, onion, Brussels sprouts, and wine to the other side.
5. Roast within 8 minutes. Remove, and let rest for 5 minutes.
6. Sprinkle with the lemon juice and serve.

Nutrition: Calories: 416 Total Fat: 27g Total Carbohydrates: 8g Sugar: 2g Fiber: 3g Protein: 22g Sodium: 636mg

27. Miso Salmon and Green Beans

Preparation Time: 10 minutes
Cooking Time: 25 minutes
Servings: 4
Ingredients:
- 1 tablespoon sesame oil
- 1-pound green beans, trimmed
- 1-pound skin-on salmon fillets, cut into 4 steaks
- ¼ cup white miso
- 2 teaspoons gluten-free tamari or soy sauce
- 2 scallions, thinly sliced

Directions:
1. Preheat the oven to 400°F. Grease the baking sheet with the oil.
2. Put the green beans, then the salmon on top of the green beans, and brush each piece with the miso.
3. Roast within 20 to 25 minutes.
4. Drizzle with the tamari, sprinkle with the scallions, and serve.

Nutrition: Calories: 213 Total Fat: 7g Total Carbohydrates: 13g Sugar: 3g Fiber: 5g Protein: 27g Sodium: 989mg

28. Tilapia with Asparagus and Acorn Squash

Preparation Time: 15 minutes
Cooking Time: 30 minutes
Servings: 4

Ingredients:

- 2 tablespoons extra-virgin olive oil
- 1 medium acorn squash, seeded and thinly sliced or in wedges
- 1-pound asparagus, trimmed of woody ends and cut into 2-inch pieces
- 1 large shallot, thinly sliced
- 1-pound tilapia fillets
- ½ cup white wine
- 1 tablespoon chopped fresh flat-leaf parsley
- 1 teaspoon salt
- ¼ teaspoon freshly ground black pepper

Directions:

1. Preheat the oven to 400°F. Grease the baking sheet with the oil.
2. Arrange the squash, asparagus, and shallot in a single layer on the baking sheet. Roast within 8 to 10 minutes.
3. Put the tilapia, and add the wine.
4. Sprinkle with the parsley, salt, and pepper.
5. Roast within 15 minutes. Remove, then let rest for 5 minutes, and serve.

Nutrition: Calories: 246 Total Fat: 8g Total Carbohydrates: 17g Sugar: 2g Fiber: 4g Protein: 25g Sodium: 639mg

29. Shrimp-Lime Bake with Zucchini and Corn

Preparation Time: 10 minutes
Cooking Time: 20 minutes
Servings: 4

Ingredients:

- 1 tablespoon extra-virgin olive oil
- 2 small zucchinis, cut into ¼-inch dice
- 1 cup frozen corn kernels
- 2 scallions, thinly sliced
- 1 teaspoon salt
- ½ teaspoon ground cumin
- ½ teaspoon chipotle chili powder
- 1-pound peeled shrimp, thawed if necessary
- 1 tablespoon finely chopped fresh cilantro
- Zest and juice of 1 lime

Directions:

1. Preheat the oven to 400°F. Grease the baking sheet with the oil.
2. On the baking sheet, combine the zucchini, corn, scallions, salt, cumin, and chile powder and mix well. Arrange in a single layer.
3. Add the shrimp on top. Roast within 15 to 20 minutes.
4. Put the cilantro and lime zest and juice, stir to combine, and serve.

Nutrition: Calories: 184 Total Fat: 5g Total Carbohydrates: 11g Sugar: 3g Fiber: 2g Protein: 26g Sodium: 846mg

30. Broccolini with Almonds

Preparation Time: 15 minutes
Cooking Time: 5 minutes
Servings: 6
Ingredients:

- 1 fresh red chili, deseeded and finely chopped
- 2 bunches of broccolini, trimmed
- 1 tablespoon extra-virgin olive oil
- 2 garlic cloves, thinly sliced
- 1/4 cup natural almonds, coarsely chopped
- 2 teaspoons lemon rind, finely grated
- 4 anchovies in oil, chopped
- A squeeze of fresh lemon juice

Directions:

1. Preheat some oil in a pan. Add 2 teaspoons of lemon rind, drained anchovies, finely chopped chili, and thinly sliced gloves. Cook for about 30 seconds, with constant stirring.
2. Add 1/4 cup coarsely chopped almonds and cook for a minute. Turn the heat off and add lemon juice on top.
3. Place the steamer basket over a pan with simmering water. Add broccolini to a basket and cover it.
4. Cook until tender-crisp, for about 3-4 minutes. Drain and then transfer to the serving platter.
5. Top with almond mixture and enjoy!

Nutrition: 414 calories 6.6 g fat 1.6 g total carbs 5.4 g protein

31. Vegetable and Chicken Stir Fry

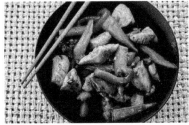

Preparation Time: 5 minutes
Cooking Time: 15 minutes
Servings: 6

Ingredients:

- 3 tablespoons of olive oil
- 3 chicken breasts
- 3 medium zucchini or yellow squash
- 2 onions
- 1 teaspoon of garlic powder
- 1 broccoli
- 1 teaspoon basil
- 1 teaspoon of pepper and salt

Directions:

1. Chop the vegetables and chicken.
2. Heat your skillet over medium temperature.
3. Pour olive oil and add the chicken. Cook while stirring.
4. Include the seasonings if you want.
5. Add the vegetables. Keep cooking until it gets slightly soft. Add the onions first and broccoli last.

Nutrition Calories 183 Carbohydrates 9g Cholesterol 41mg Total Fat 11g Protein 12g Sugar 4g Fiber 3g Sodium 468mg

SIDE DISHES

32. Oregano Green Beans

Preparation time: 10 minutes
Cooking time: 15 minutes
Servings: 4
Ingredients:
- 1-pound green beans, trimmed and halved
- 1 cup of water
- 1 tablespoon dried oregano
- 1 teaspoon chili powder
- 1 tablespoon almond butter

Directions:
1. Bring the water to boil.
2. Add green beans and boil them for 10 minutes.
3. Then transfer the green beans in the bowl and add dried oregano, chili powder, and almond butter.
4. Stir the meal well.

Nutrition: 65 calories, 3.1g protein, 9.9g carbohydrates, 2.6g fat, 5g fiber, 0mg cholesterol, 16mg sodium, 299mg potassium.

33. Guacamole Salad

Preparation Time: 10 minutes
Cooking Time: 0 minutes
Servings: 4
Ingredients:
- 2 avocados, cut into 1-inch chunks
- 4 Roma tomatoes, quartered
- 1 green bell pepper, cut into 1-inch chunks
- ¼ red onion, thinly sliced
- ½ cup packed whole fresh cilantro leaves
- ¼ cup extra-virgin olive oil
- Juice of 2 limes
- 1 teaspoon salt
- ½ teaspoon freshly ground black pepper

Directions:
1. In a medium bowl, combine the avocados, tomatoes, bell pepper, onion, and cilantro.
2. In a small bowl, whisk together the olive oil, lime juice, salt, and pepper and drizzle over the salad. Toss to coat well and serve immediately.

Nutrition: Calories: 258; Total Fat: 24g; Total Carbs: 12g; Net Carbs: 6g; Fiber: 6g; Protein: 2g; Sodium: 600mg; Macros: Fat: 84%, Carbs: 13%, Protein: 3%

34. Curried Tuna Salad with Pepitas

Preparation Time: 10 minutes
Cooking Time: 0 minutes
Servings: 2
Ingredients:

- 1 ripe avocado, halved and pitted
- Juice of 1 lime
- 1 tablespoon avocado or extra-virgin olive oil
- 1 teaspoon curry powder
- ½ teaspoon salt
- 1 (4-ounce) can olive oil–packed tuna
- 2 tablespoons chopped fresh cilantro
- 2 tablespoons roasted pumpkin seeds

Directions:

1. Using a spoon, scoop the avocado flesh into a medium bowl and mash well with a fork.
2. Add the lime juice, avocado oil, curry powder, and salt and mix well. Add the tuna and its oil, cilantro, and pumpkin seeds and mix well with a fork.
3. Eat immediately or store covered in the refrigerator for up to three days.

Nutrition: Calories: 347; Total Fat: 26g; Total Carbs: 9g; Net Carbs: 3g; Fiber: 6g; Protein: 22g; Sodium: 854mg; Macros: Fat: 67%, Carbs: 8%, Protein: 25%

35. Moroccan-Spiced Cauliflower Salad

Preparation Time: 5 minutes
Cooking Time: 25 minutes, plus 15 minutes to cool
Servings: 4

Ingredients:

- 4 cups fresh or frozen cauliflower florets
- 2 tablespoons coconut oil, melted
- 1 teaspoon salt, divided
- ¼ cup extra-virgin olive oil
- Grated zest and juice of 1 lemon
- 1 teaspoon chili powder
- 1 teaspoon ground cinnamon
- 1 teaspoon garlic powder
- ½ teaspoon ground turmeric
- ½ teaspoon ground ginger
- 2 celery stalks, thinly sliced
- ½ cup finely sliced fresh mint
- ¼ cup finely sliced red onion
- ¼ cup shelled pistachios

Directions:

1. If using frozen cauliflower, thaw to room temperature in a colander, draining off any excess water. Cut larger florets into bite-size pieces.
2. Preheat the oven to 450°F and line a baking sheet with aluminum foil.
3. In a medium bowl, toss the cauliflower with coconut oil and ½ teaspoon of salt. Arrange the cauliflower in a single layer on the prepared baking sheet, reserving the seasoned bowl.
4. Roast the cauliflower for 20 to 25 minutes, until it is lightly browned and crispy.

5. While the cauliflower roasts, in the reserved bowl, whisk together the olive oil, lemon zest and juice, the remaining ½ teaspoon of salt, the chili powder, cinnamon, garlic powder, turmeric, and ginger. Stir in the celery, mint, and onion.
6. When the cauliflower is done roasting, remove from the oven and allow to cool for 10 to 15 minutes.
7. Toss the warm (but not too hot) cauliflower with the dressing until well combined. Add the pistachios and toss to incorporate. Serve warm or chilled.

Nutrition: Calories: 262; Total Fat: 24g; Total Carbs: 11g; Net Carbs: 7g; Fiber: 4g; Protein: 4g; Sodium: 651mg; Macros: Fat: 82%, Carbs: 12%, Protein: 6%

36. Creamy Riced Cauliflower Salad

Preparation Time: 10 minutes, plus 30 minutes to chill
Cooking Time: 0 minutes
Servings: 4
Ingredients:

- 4 ounces crumbled sheep's milk feta cheese
- ½ cup Anti-Inflammatory Mayo
- Grated zest and juice of 1 lemon
- 2 tablespoons minced red onion
- 1½ teaspoons dried dill
- ½ teaspoon salt
- 1 teaspoon red pepper flakes, or to taste
- 3 cups fresh riced cauliflower (not frozen)
- ½ cup coarsely chopped pitted Kalamata olives

Directions:

1. In a medium bowl, combine the feta, mayo, lemon zest and juice, onion, dill, salt, and red pepper flakes. Whisk well with a fork until smooth and creamy.
2. Add the cauliflower and olives and mix well to combine.
3. Refrigerate for at least 30 minutes before serving.

Nutrition: Calories: 370; Total Fat: 37g; Total Carbs: 6g; Net Carbs: 4g; Fiber: 2g; Protein: 7g; Sodium: 1048mg; Macros: Fat: 90%, Carbs: 2%, Protein: 8%

37. Weekday Omega-3 Salad

Preparation Time: 10 minutes
Cooking Time: 0 minutes
Servings: 2

Ingredients:

- 6 cups baby arugula or spinach
- 1 (4-ounce) can olive oil–packed tuna, mackerel, or salmon
- ¼ cup minced fresh parsley
- 10 green or black olives, pitted and halved
- 2 tablespoons minced scallions, white and green parts, or red onion
- 1 avocado, thinly sliced
- ¼ cup roasted pumpkin or sunflower seeds
- 6 tablespoons Basic Vinaigrette or Caesar Dressing

Directions:

1. Divide the greens between bowls.
2. In a small bowl, combine the tuna and its oil with the parsley, olives, and scallions. Divide the fish mixture evenly on top of the greens.
3. Divide the avocado slices and pumpkin seeds between the bowls. Drizzle each with the dressing and toss to coat.

Nutrition: Calories: 716; Total Fat: 61g; Total Carbs: 16g; Net Carbs: 5g; Fiber: 11g; Protein: 31g; Sodium: 1021mg; Macros: Fat: 77%, Carbs: 6%, Protein: 17%

38. Classic Coleslaw

Preparation Time: 15 minutes, plus 30 minutes to chill
Cooking Time: 0 minutes
Servings: 4
Ingredients:
- ½ cup Anti-Inflammatory Mayo
- 1 tablespoon avocado or extra-virgin olive oil
- 1 tablespoon Dijon mustard
- 1 tablespoon freshly squeezed lemon juice or apple cider vinegar
- 1 teaspoon salt
- ½ teaspoon ground turmeric
- ½ teaspoon freshly ground black pepper
- 3 cups shredded green cabbage
- 1 cup shredded red cabbage
- 1 cup coarsely chopped baby spinach leaves
- ½ cup chopped fresh cilantro, basil, or parsley
- ¼ small red onion, thinly sliced
- ¼ cup roasted pumpkin seeds or slivered almonds

Directions:
1. In a small bowl, whisk together the mayo, avocado oil, mustard, lemon juice, salt, turmeric, and pepper. Set aside.
2. In a large bowl, combine the green and red cabbages, spinach, cilantro, and red onion. Add the dressing and toss to coat well. Refrigerate for at least 30 minutes to allow flavors to develop.
3. Serve chilled, topped with the pumpkin seeds.

Nutrition: Calories: 349; Total Fat: 35g; Total Carbs: 7g; Net Carbs: 4g; Fiber: 3g; Protein: 4g; Sodium: 856mg; Macros: Fat: 90%, Carbs: 5%, Protein: 5%

39. Weeknight Greek Salad

Preparation Time: 5 minutes
Cooking Time: 0 minutes
Servings: 4

Ingredients:

- 8 cups coarsely chopped romaine lettuce
- 4 ounces crumbled sheep's milk feta cheese
- ½ cup Marinated Antipasto Veggies or store-bought marinated artichoke hearts
- 20 Kalamata olives, pitted
- 2 tablespoons chopped fresh oregano or rosemary, or 2 teaspoons dried oregano
- ¼ cup extra-virgin olive oil
- Juice of 1 lemon
- ½ teaspoon freshly ground black pepper

Directions:

1. In a large bowl, combine the lettuce, feta, antipasto veggies, olives, and oregano. Drizzle with the olive oil, then add the lemon juice and pepper. Toss to coat and serve immediately.

Nutrition: Calories: 300; Total Fat: 27g; Total Carbs: 10g; Net Carbs: 7g; Fiber: 3g; Protein: 6g; Sodium: 795mg; Macros: Fat: 81%, Carbs: 11%, Protein: 8%

40. <u>Italian Green Bean Salad</u>

Preparation Time: 5 minutes
Cooking Time: 5 minutes, plus 1 hour to chill
Servings: 4

Ingredients:

- ¼ cup extra-virgin olive oil, divided
- 1-pound green beans, trimmed
- 2 tablespoons red wine vinegar
- 1 teaspoon salt
- 1 teaspoon red pepper flakes
- 2 garlic cloves, thinly sliced
- ½ cup slivered almonds
- ¼ cup thinly sliced fresh basil
- 2 tablespoons chopped fresh mint

Directions:

1. In a large skillet, heat 2 tablespoons of olive oil over medium-high heat. Add the green beans and sauté for about 5 minutes, until they are just tender. Remove from the heat and transfer to a large serving bowl.
2. In a small bowl, whisk together the remaining 2 tablespoons of olive oil, the vinegar, salt, red pepper flakes, and garlic. Pour the dressing over the green beans and toss to coat well.
3. Add the almonds, basil, and mint and toss well. Serve warm or chill for at least 1 hour to serve cold.

Nutrition: Calories: 238; Total Fat: 21g; Total Carbs: 12g; Net Carbs: 7g; Fiber: 5g; Protein: 5g; Sodium: 598mg; Macros: Fat: 79%, Carbs: 13%, Protein: 8

MEAT

41. Beef with Carrot & Broccoli

Preparation Time: 15 minutes
Cooking Time: 14 minutes
Servings: 4

Ingredients:

- ¼ cup chicken broth
- ¼ tsp. freshly ground black pepper
- ½ tsp. Red pepper flakes, crushed
- 1 big carrot, peeled and cut thinly
- 1 lb. beef sirloin steak, cut into fine strips
- 1 medium scallion, cut thinly
- 1 tbsp. Ground flax seeds
- 2 cups broccoli florets
- 2 medium garlic cloves, minced
- 2 tbsp. coconut oil, divided
- 2 tsp. fresh ginger, grated
- Salt, to taste

Directions:

1. In a frying pan, warm 1 tbsp. of oil on moderate to high heat.
2. Put garlic and sauté roughly one minute.
3. Put in beef and salt and cook for minimum 4-5 minutes or till browned.
4. Use a slotted spoon to move the beef in a container.
5. Take off the liquid from the frying pan.
6. In a container, put together broth, ginger, flax seeds, red pepper flakes, and black pepper then mix.

7. In the same frying pan, warm remaining oil on moderate heat.
8. Place the carrot, broccoli, and ginger mixture then cook for minimum 3-4 minutes or till desired doneness.
9. Stir in beef and scallion then cook for about four minutes.

Nutrition: Calories: 412, Fat: 13g, Carbohydrates: 28g, Fiber: 9g, Protein: 35g

42. Beef with Mushroom & Broccoli

Preparation Time: 15 minutes
Cooking Time: twelve minutes
Servings: 4
Ingredients:
For Beef Marinade:

- ¾ cup beef broth
- 1 (2-inch piece fresh ginger, minced
- 1 garlic clove, minced
- 1 lb. flank steak, trimmed and cut into fine strips
- 3 tbsp. white wine vinegar
- Freshly ground black pepper, to taste
- Salt, to taste

For Vegetables:

- 2 minced garlic cloves
- 2 tbsp. coconut oil, divided
- 3 cups broccoli rabe, chopped
- 4 oz. shiitake mushrooms halved
- 8 oz. cremini mushrooms, cut

Directions:

1. For marinade in a container, put together all ingredients apart from beef then mix.
2. Put in beef and coat with marinade.
3. Bring in your refrigerator to marinate for minimum fifteen minutes.
4. In the frying pan, warm oil on moderate to high heat.
5. Take off beef from the container, saving for later the marinade.
6. Put beef and garlic and cook for approximately 3-4 minutes or till browned.
7. Use a slotted spoon to move the beef in a container.

8. In the same frying pan, put the reserved marinade, broccoli, and mushrooms and cook for minimum 3-4 minutes.
9. Mix in beef and cook for minimum 3-4 minutes.

Nutrition: Calories: 417, Fat: 10g, Carbohydrates: 23g, Fiber: 11g, Protein: 33g

43. Beef with Zucchini Noodles

Preparation Time: 15 minutes
Cooking Time: 9 minutes
Servings: 4
Ingredients:

- ¼ cup coconut aminos
- 1 teaspoon fresh ginger, grated
- 1 teaspoon red pepper flakes, crushed
- 1½ pound NY strip steak, trimmed and cut thinly
- 2 medium garlic cloves, minced
- 2 medium scallions, cut
- 2 medium zucchinis, spiralized with Blade C
- 2 tablespoons fresh cilantro, chopped
- 2 tablespoons fresh lime juice
- 3 tablespoons essential olive oil
- Salt, to taste

Directions:

1. In a big container, combine ginger, garlic, coconut aminos, and lime juice.
2. Put in beef and coat with marinade liberally.
3. Place in your fridge to marinate for roughly ten minutes.
4. Put zucchini noodles over a big paper towel and drizzle with salt.
5. Keep aside for around ten minutes.
6. In a big frying pan, heat oil on moderate to high heat.
7. Put in scallion and red pepper flakes and sauté for approximately one minute.
8. Put in beef with marinade and stir fry for about four minutes or till browned.
9. Put in zucchini and cook for roughly 3-4 minutes.

10. Serve hot with all the topping of cilantro.

Nutrition: Calories: 434, Fat: 17g, Carbohydrates: 23g, Fiber: 12g, Protein: 29g

44. Berry Chops Dinner

Preparation Time: ten minutes
Cooking Time: 15 minutes
Servings: 4
Ingredients:
- (ground) black pepper and salt to taste
- ½ cup balsamic vinegar
- ½ teaspoon thyme, dried
- 1 teaspoon cinnamon powder
- 12 ounces blackberries
- 2 pounds pork chops
- 2 tablespoons water

Directions:
1. Spice the pork chops with salt, pepper, cinnamon, and thyme.
2. Heat up a cooking pot; put in the blackberries and heat on moderate heat.
3. Put in the vinegar, water, salt, and pepper, stir the mix.
4. Simmer for three to five minutes and take it off the heat.
5. Brush the pork chops with half of the blueberry mix.
6. Preheat your grill and grill the chops on moderate heat for about six minutes on each side.
7. Split the pork chops between serving plates; top with the remaining blackberry sauce. Serve warm.

Nutrition: Calories 286 , Fat: 6g , Carbohydrates: 11g , Fiber: 6g , Protein: 22g

45. Cauliflower Lamb Meal

Preparation Time: five minutes
Cooking Time: 20 minutes
Servings: 4
Ingredients:
Mash:

- ½ teaspoon garlic powder
- ½ teaspoon salt
- 1 big head cauliflower, cut into florets
- Dash cayenne pepper
- Lamb:
- ½ teaspoon freshly ground black pepper
- 1 teaspoon dried rosemary
- 1 teaspoon salt
- 2 (8-ounce) grass-fed lamb fillets
- 2 tablespoons avocado oil

Directions:

1. In cooking (you can also use a deep cooking pan), put in the cauliflower and water to immerse it.
2. Heat it over the medium stove flame. Boil and cook for about ten minutes. Drain water and move the cauliflower to a food processor (or blender).
3. Put in the ghee, garlic powder, salt, and cayenne pepper. Blend until smooth.
4. Spice the lamb with the pepper and salt.
5. In a frying pan or deep cooking pan, warm the oil on the medium stove flame.
6. Put in the lamb, rosemary, and cook, while stirring, until it becomes uniformly brown for 8-ten minutes.
7. Cut the lamb into coins and serve with the cauliflower mash.

Nutrition: Calories 294 , Fat: 17g , Carbohydrates: 11g , Fiber: 3g , Protein: 36g

46. Italian Meatballs in Asiago Sauce

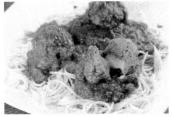

Preparation time: 15 minutes
Cooking time: 15 minutes
Servings: 3

Ingredients

- 1 teaspoon Italian spice mix
- 1/2 pound ground beef
- 1 egg
- 3 ounces Asiago cheese, grated
- 1/4 cup mayonnaise

Directions

1. In a mixing bowl, thoroughly combine Italian slice mix, beef, and egg. Mix until everything is well combined. Roll the mixture into meatballs.
2. In another bowl, mix Asiago cheese and mayonnaise.
3. Heat 1 tablespoon of olive oil in a frying pan over a moderate heat. Then, sear the meatballs for about 5 minutes, turning them occasionally to ensure even cooking. Bon appétit!

Nutrition: 458 Calories; 35.8g Fat; 4.3g Carbs; 28.2g Protein; 0.2g Fiber

47. Meatloaf with a Sweet Sticky Glaze

Preparation Time: 1 hour
Cooking Time: 70 minutes
Servings: 2
Ingredients

- 3/4 pound ground chuck
- 1/4 cup flaxseed meal
- 2 eggs, beaten
- 1/2 cup tomato sauce with garlic and onion
- 1 teaspoon liquid monk fruit

Directions

1. In a mixing bowl, combine the ground chuck, flaxseed meal, and eggs; season with the salt and black pepper.
2. In a separate mixing bowl, combine the tomato sauce and liquid monk fruit; add 1 teaspoon of mustard and whisk until well combined.
3. Spoon the mixture into the foil-lined loaf pan and smooth the surface. Bake in the preheated oven at 365 degrees F for about 25 minutes.
4. Spoon the tomato mixture on top of the meatloaf and continue to bake for a further 25 minutes or until thoroughly cooked.
5. Allow your meatloaf to rest for 10 minutes before slicing and. Bon appétit!

Nutrition: 517 Calories; 32.3g Fat; 8.4g Carbs; 48.5g Protein; 6.5g Fiber

48. Pork Chops with Shallots

Preparation Time: 10 minutes
Cooking Time: 40 minutes
Servings: 4
Ingredients:
- 1 cup shallots, chopped
- ½ cup vegetable stock
- 2 pounds pork stew meat, roughly cubed
- 2 garlic cloves, minced
- A pinch of salt and black pepper
- 2 tablespoons olive oil
- 1 tablespoon cilantro, chopped

Directions:
1. Heat up a pan with the oil over medium-high heat, add the shallots and sauté for 10 minutes.
2. Add the meat and the other ingredients, toss, cook over medium heat for 30 minutes, divide between plates and serve.

Nutrition: calories 250, fat 12, fiber 2, carbs 13, protein 17

49. Mint Pork

Preparation Time: 10 minutes
Cooking Time: 40 minutes
Servings: 4
Ingredients:

- 4 pork chops
- 1 cup mint leaves
- 2 tablespoons balsamic vinegar
- 1 tablespoon almonds, chopped
- 2 tablespoons olive oil
- 2 garlic cloves, minced
- Salt and black pepper to the taste
- ¼ teaspoon red pepper flakes

Directions:

1. In a blender, combine the mint with the vinegar and the other ingredients except the pork chops and pulse well.
2. Heat up a pan with the mint mix over medium heat, add the pork chops, toss, introduce in the oven and bake at 390 degrees F for 40 minutes.
3. Divide everything between plates and serve.

Nutrition: calories 260, fat 6 fiber 1, carbs 8, protein 23

50. Pork with Spiced Zucchinis

Preparation Time: 10 minutes
Cooking Time: 40 minutes
Servings: 4

Ingredients:
- 2 pounds pork stew meat, roughly cubed
- 2 zucchinis, sliced
- 2 tablespoons olive oil
- 1 teaspoon nutmeg, ground
- 1 teaspoon cinnamon powder
- 1 teaspoon cumin, ground
- 2 tablespoons lime juice
- 2 garlic cloves, minced
- A pinch of sea salt and black pepper

Directions:
1. In a roasting pan, combine the meat with the zucchinis, the nutmeg and the other ingredients, toss and bake at 390 degrees F for 40 minutes.
2. Divide everything between plates and serve.

Nutrition: calories 200, fat 5, fiber 2, carbs 10, protein 22

CPSIA information can be obtained
at www.ICGtesting.com
Printed in the USA
LVHW011641130621
690126LV00014B/1082